# THE
# HEART AND BLOOD

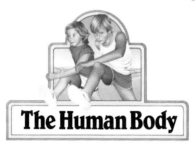

The Human Body

# THE
# HEART AND BLOOD

Brian R. Ward

Series consultant:
**Dr A. R. Maryon-Davis**
MB, B.Chir, MSc, MRCS, MRCP

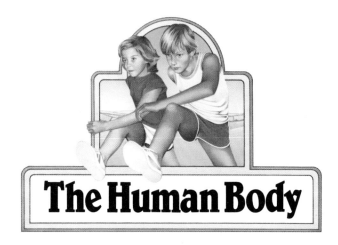

**The Human Body**

**Franklin Watts**
London New York Sydney Toronto

Franklin Watts Inc.

6.2.82

First published in Great Britain in 1982 by
Franklin Watts Limited
8 Cork Street
London W1

First published in the United States of America by
Franklin Watts Inc.
730 Fifth Avenue
New York
N.Y. 10019

UK ISBN: 0 85166 945 X
US ISBN: 0-531-04357-6
Library of Congress Catalog Card No: 81-51679

Designed by Howard Dyke

Phototypeset by Computape (Pickering) Ltd, North Yorkshire
Printed in Great Britain by E. T. Heron, London and Essex

**Acknowledgments**

The illustrations were prepared by: Andrew Aloof, Bob
Chapman, Howard Dyke, Hayward Art Group, David Holmes,
David Mallott.

# Contents

# Introduction

The **heart** and the **circulation** of the **blood** form one of the most important transport systems in the body. The heart is a pump which forces blood through a network of tubes, or blood vessels, throughout the whole body.

As it travels through the body, blood carries out several essential jobs. It carries life-giving **oxygen** to nearly all the cells of the body, and removes waste materials produced by body activity. Food materials needed for cell growth, and to maintain the cells, are also carried in the bloodstream. Other vital materials present in the blood are chemical messengers called **hormones**, which act on various parts of the body, and **antibodies**, chemicals which fight disease.

In an adult, the whole system contains 10 to 12 pints (5–6 liters) of blood, and makes up about a twelfth of the body's weight.

The blood circulates through a huge network of blood vessels, some of which are so fine that, if all the tubes in the blood system were laid end to end, there would be more than 100,000 miles (160,000 km) of blood vessels.

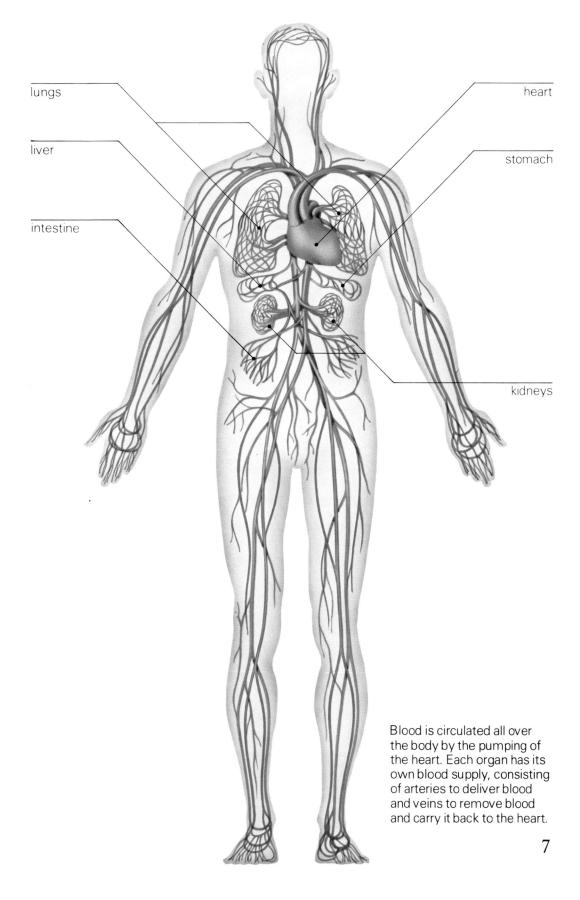

lungs

liver

intestine

heart

stomach

kidneys

Blood is circulated all over the body by the pumping of the heart. Each organ has its own blood supply, consisting of arteries to deliver blood and veins to remove blood and carry it back to the heart.

7

# The body's transport system

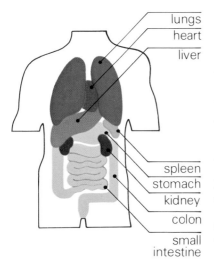

lungs
heart
liver

spleen
stomach
kidney
colon
small intestine

Each of the major organs of the body has a special blood supply.

Each of the billions of living cells that make up the body needs oxygen and food in order to live, and these are supplied by the blood. This means that blood must be carried into every organ of the body, so that each cell can obtain the oxygen and nourishment it needs.

A network of tiny branched tubes carrying the blood runs through the brain, skin, muscle and every other part of the body. These tubes, called **capillaries**, are normally only absent from non-living parts of the body, like the fingernails and hair.

Blood is supplied to the capillaries by much larger vessels called **arteries**, and drains out into other large vessels called **veins**. Blood is pumped around the system by the heart, never ceasing its flow and never leaking out except when we are injured.

The circulatory system consists of two parts. First the blood is pumped from the heart, around the body, and is returned to the heart. At this stage, oxygen has been used up, and waste materials like **carbon dioxide** ($CO_2$) have entered the bloodstream. But, instead of being pumped back around the body, the blood is now pumped to the lungs, where oxygen is replaced and $CO_2$ removed. Then the blood is pumped back to the heart and around the body to begin the cycle again.

Blood follows a doubled course around the body. It passes through the lungs, back to the heart, and is pumped around the body before returning to the heart and beginning its journey again.

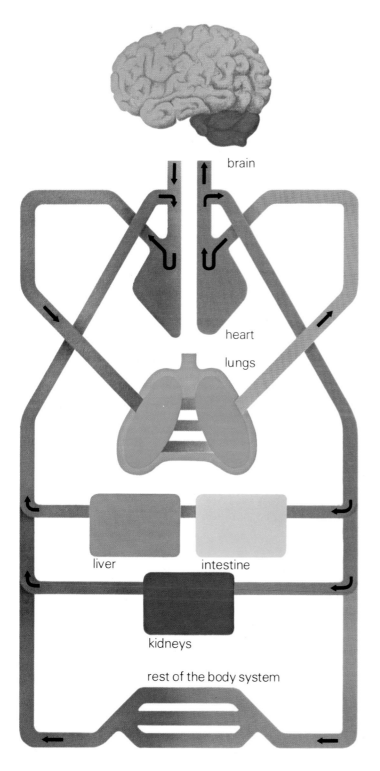

brain

heart

lungs

liver

intestine

kidneys

rest of the body system

# The structure of the heart

The heart consists of two powerful pump units, each with an upper and lower chamber and with valves to prevent blood from flowing backward as it pumps.

The heart is made up almost entirely of muscle. It is a large, tough organ, about the size of a clenched fist. It is positioned on the center line of the body, about halfway down the chest, just beneath the breastbone. It is tilted so that the lower end points toward the left.

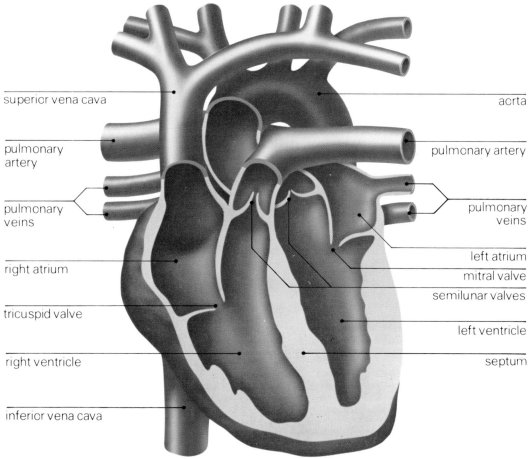

superior vena cava

aorta

pulmonary artery

pulmonary artery

pulmonary veins

pulmonary veins

left atrium

right atrium

mitral valve

semilunar valves

tricuspid valve

left ventricle

right ventricle

septum

inferior vena cava

The heart is basically a pump. One that works well can operate for sixty to a hundred years or more. The heart is made up of four distinct chambers. The entire four-chambered pump is surrounded by a protective layer called the **pericardium**, which contains a lubricating liquid.

The four chambers of the heart consist of two upper chambers and two lower chambers. The upper chambers are thin walled and they receive blood returning to the heart from the large veins of the body. These chambers are called the left **atrium** and the right atrium (plural, atria).

The lower chambers of the heart are called the left and right **ventricles**. They are much larger and very much more muscular than the atria. The right ventricle pumps blood to the lungs and the left ventricle pumps blood to the rest of the body.

The left and right sides of the heart are divided by a tough wall called the **septum**. This thick wall separates the blood which is to be pumped to the lungs from the blood which will go to the rest of the body. Blood is kept moving in the proper direction by a series of valves. These are leathery flaps which are forced open by the pressure of blood and then shut to stop it draining back.

The heart is equipped with a series of one-way valves to keep blood flowing in the proper direction. These are small flaps, made of tough, rubbery material, which are forced open by the passage of blood.

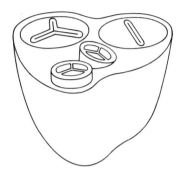

Semilunar valves prevent blood from flowing back into the heart from the aorta and pulmonary artery.

Mitral or bicuspid valve opens to allow blood to leave the left atrium and enter the ventricle.

Tricuspid valve opens to allow blood to leave the right atrium and enter the ventricle.

# How the heart pumps

It is very important that "fresh" or oxygenated blood is kept separate from "stale" or deoxygenated blood that has already been passed around the body.

Blood returning to the heart from the body, laden with $CO_2$, and containing little oxygen, first enters the right atrium, at the top of the heart. The atrium contracts gently, squeezing the blood through a one-way valve into the right ventricle, immediately below.

The right ventricle contracts powerfully, pumping the blood along arteries to the lungs, where oxygen is replenished and $CO_2$ is removed. Oxygenated blood returns from the lungs to the left atrium, and is in turn pumped through another valve into the left ventricle. The left ventricle is the most powerful part of the heart's pump mechanism, and when it contracts, it forces blood all around the body.

To summarize, the blood circulation passes from the heart to the lungs, and back to the heart. Then it travels around the body, and back to the heart once more.

Occasionally, a baby is born with a small hole in the septum dividing the right and left sides of the heart, allowing oxygenated and deoxygenated blood to mix. Surgery is needed to correct this "hole in the heart."

1 Oxygenated blood from the lungs (red) enters the left atrium. At the same time deoxygenated blood (blue) returns from being pumped around the body to the right atrium.

2 Both atria contract, opening their valves and forcing blood into the ventricles.

3 As the ventricles begin to contract, the atrial valves close.

4 The ventricles force blood out of the heart, to the lungs and around the body.

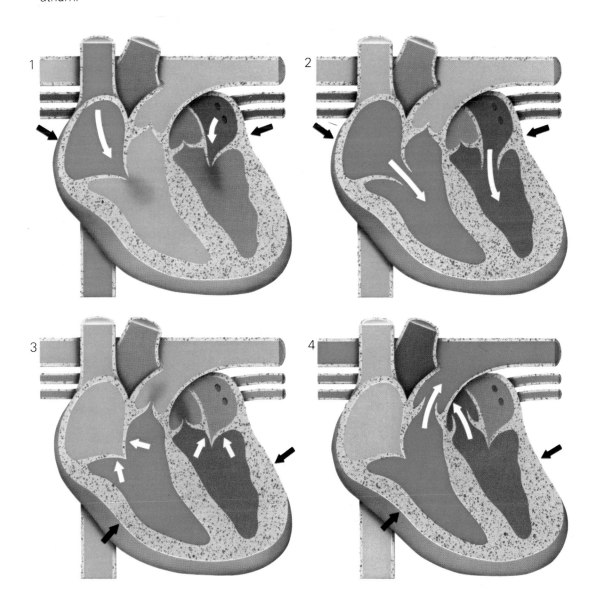

# Timing the heart

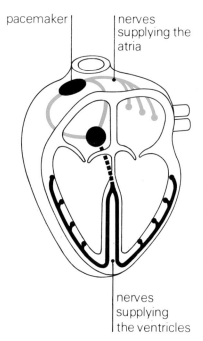

pacemaker | nerves supplying the atria

nerves supplying the ventricles

The heart's pacemaker generates the regular electrical signals which cause the heart to pump. Its signals first cause the atria to contract, followed a moment later by the contraction of the ventricles.

The heart is made up from a special type of muscle, called **cardiac muscle**. Like other muscle, it consists of threads or muscle fibers which contract to produce movement, but it is unusual in that the fibers are branched and connected in a dense network.

This means that when one muscle fiber in the heart contracts, the chemical changes within it can spread through the branched network so that all the connected fibers contract at roughly the same time. Since the heart's chambers are hollow, this contraction causes the blood they contain to be squeezed out into the connecting arteries.

The heart beats, or contracts, regularly, and must continue to do so in order to maintain the blood flow. Several types of control keep the heart beating steadily.

The heart has its own timing mechanism, in the wall of the right atrium. This tiny patch of cells produces nerve impulses at regular intervals which tell the heart muscle to contract, starting with the atria, followed soon after by contraction of the ventricles. The timing signal is produced within the heart and works even after a living heart has been transplanted. The electrical signals can be recorded, traced and studied using a machine which produces an **electrocardiogram**.

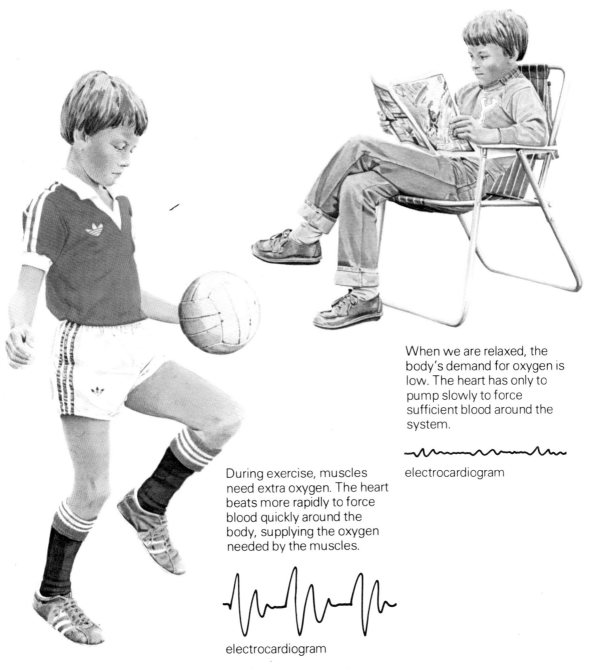

During exercise, muscles need extra oxygen. The heart beats more rapidly to force blood quickly around the body, supplying the oxygen needed by the muscles.

electrocardiogram

When we are relaxed, the body's demand for oxygen is low. The heart has only to pump slowly to force sufficient blood around the system.

electrocardiogram

The nervous system can speed up or slow down the rate at which the heart beats, as, for instance, when we are excited, or asleep. Yet another mechanism measures the level of oxygen and $CO_2$, and varies the rate at which the heart beats in order to keep these gases at their proper levels in the blood.

# The pulse

Each contraction of the powerful left ventricle sends a jet of blood into the arteries. The blood is under pressure, so each pumping action causes the flexible wall of the artery to bulge slightly. The blood then squeezes through narrow capillaries before reaching the veins. This helps to smooth out the pumping action so that the blood now flows evenly.

The bulging of the arteries with each beat of the heart is the pulse. It can be seen and felt with the fingertips where arteries lie just beneath the skin, particularly at the side of the neck, the inside of the wrist and the back of the knee. By placing a fingertip on the inside of the wrist, on the side nearest the thumb, a pulse can be felt. This corresponds to the contractions of the left ventricle.

A similar pulse can be felt in the center of the chest, but this is caused by the movement of the heart muscle.

The doctor places a **stethoscope** over the heart to listen to heart sounds, which are caused by the opening and closing of the heart valves, and by the flowing blood. These usually sound like "lup-dup, lub-dup." If there is a fault in the heart, or if valves are not working properly, the doctor can often detect this by an alteration in the heart sounds.

Arteries flex each time the heart beats, and this can easily be felt as the pulse in the wrist. Feel for it on the inside of your wrist, on the side nearest the thumb. Use only your fingertips, as the thumb has its own pulse. A doctor or nurse often measures the pulse of a sick person, which can help in diagnosing and treating an illness.

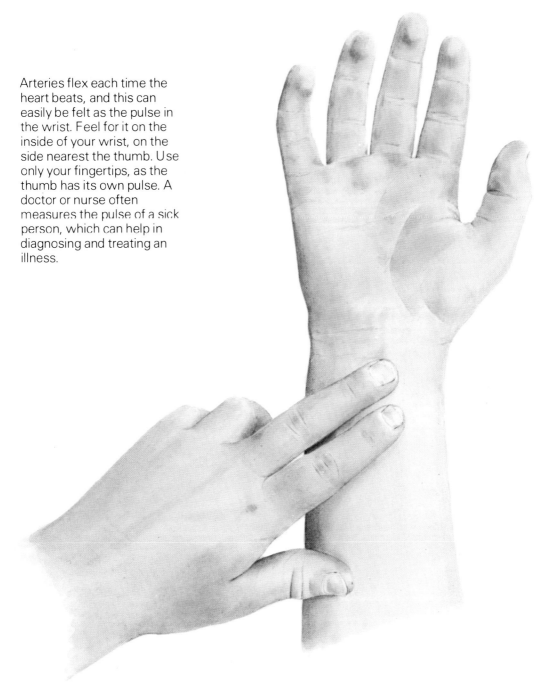

# Arteries

Arteries are the tubular blood vessels which carry blood away from the heart. Most blood is pumped into the largest vessel in the body, the **aorta**, which is about 1 inch (2·5 cm) in diameter. From the aorta, which runs down the body near the spine, branches spread to distribute blood to all the organs. The branches become finer, leading into much smaller vessels called **arterioles**.

Very large amounts of blood are pumped at high pressure into the arteries, moving at 15 inches (38 cm) per second along the aorta. Arteries need strong walls to withstand this pressure, and contain a thick layer of muscle.

As the left ventricle contracts, it forces blood out through a one-way valve into the aorta, the largest artery in the body. The jet of blood causes the aorta to bulge.

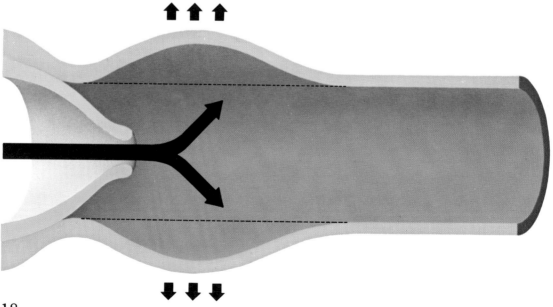

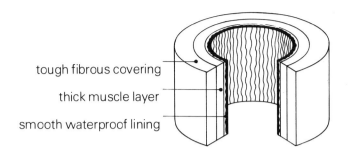

tough fibrous covering

thick muscle layer

smooth waterproof lining

The larger arteries smooth the flow of blood by expanding just after each beat of the heart, and then contracting to their normal diameter.

The walls of arterioles are even more muscular, but their function is different. They regulate the amounts of blood reaching different organs, according to the needs of the body. Arterioles can also reduce blood pressure, which might otherwise damage delicate organs.

Arteries, arterioles and veins are lined with a slippery, waterproof layer to prevent blood from leaking through their walls.

The walls of an artery contain a thick layer of muscle, which can cause it to contract.

The heart valve closes, and the muscular walls of the aorta contract to squeeze the blood along the artery on its way around the body. The contraction of the aorta comes at the right moment to help even out the jets of blood leaving the heart to produce a smooth blood flow around the body.

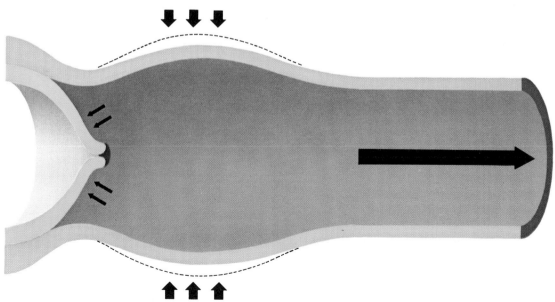

# Veins

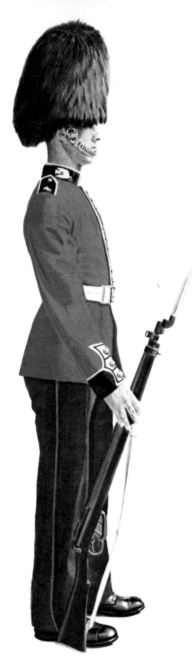

Veins return blood to the heart. They have muscle in their walls, like arteries, but are much thinner and more delicate. Blood flows through the arteries and arterioles, and then through capillaries, so that when it reaches the veins it is at low pressure. Veins bulge as the blood stretches their thin walls, and they can accommodate most of the blood in the body.

The largest veins, such as the **venae cavae**, can change their capacity by slowly contracting the muscle in their walls. This makes up for changes in the blood volume, as may be necessary after serious bleeding.

All but the smallest veins contain one-way valves that stop blood draining back in the wrong direction. Blood can collect in the veins of the legs if a person stands still for a long time. This can cause faintness, as there may not be a sufficient blood supply to the brain. Soldiers on parade are taught to keep tensing their leg muscles to squeeze blood out of the veins and allow more to reach the brain. This action takes place naturally as we move about and helps the blood to circulate.

When the valves do not work effectively, veins become swollen and painful. These can sometimes be seen as **varicose veins**, just under the skin in the legs.

In spite of the one-way valves in veins, blood sometimes collects in them when a person stands very still for a long time. This can starve the brain of blood and cause fainting. Soldiers on parade are taught to tense their leg muscles occasionally to squeeze out blood collecting in the veins.

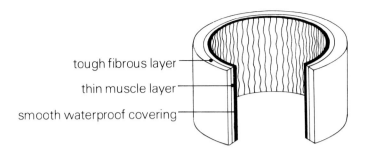

tough fibrous layer

thin muscle layer

smooth waterproof covering

In much of the body, veins are wrapped around arteries. Heat from blood in the arteries warms blood in the veins, reducing the body's heat loss. In the arms and legs, where veins are near the surface, they are not wrapped around arteries. In hot weather, blood is directed to these veins just beneath the skin, to help cool the body.

The walls of veins are thin and flexible. They contain little muscle.

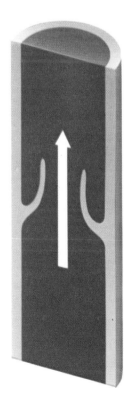 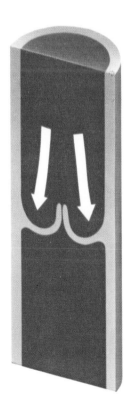

Blood passing around the body pushes its way past one-way valves in the veins.

The valves close if blood begins to flow backward. This normally prevents blood from accumulating in the legs due to its own weight.

# Capillaries

Capillaries are the smallest blood vessels in the body. Their walls are only one cell thick, and they do not have the waterproof lining found in arteries, arterioles and veins. Capillaries are so narrow that red blood cells, which are normally disc-shaped, can only just squeeze through them by being forced out of shape.

Capillaries form a complicated branched network through the whole of the body. The

Blood passes along ever-narrowing arteries and arterioles, until it enters a complicated network of fine capillaries. Eventually it finds its way back into veins, which return the blood to the heart.

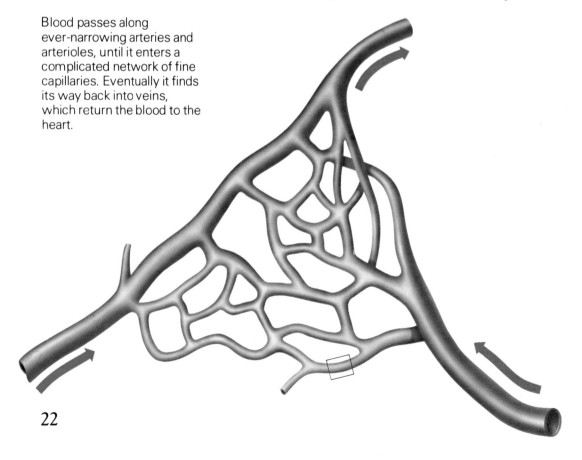

network is so immense that few cells are far away from a capillary, and all have easy access to the body's main transport system. Capillaries are the only vessels where the blood can carry out its functions of supplying oxygen and food materials and removing waste. Most chemicals can pass easily through their thin walls.

The network of capillaries in the skin gives it its normal, healthy pink color. Blood in transparent capillaries can be seen through the skin. Pinching the skin squeezes blood out of the capillaries, and the pinched area appears white. The same thing happens in cold weather, when arterioles supplying blood to the skin become narrow. This cuts off the blood supply to the capillaries, making the skin appear white or bluish in color.

Red blood cells are disc-shaped, but even these minute objects are distorted as they squeeze through the tiny capillaries. The wall of the capillary is thin and transparent, only one cell thick.

# Blood pressure

Blood is forced around the circulation by the pumping of the heart. It flows easily through healthy arteries and veins, but needs to be pushed through the microscopically narrow capillaries. Blood is a thick, sticky liquid which does not pass easily through these tiny tubes. Because of this resistance, the pressure builds up in the system of arteries as the heart continues to pump. It is highest in the arteries near the heart, and reaches a peak with each squeeze or contraction of the ventricle.

So there are actually *two* blood-pressure measurements – a high point as the ventricle pumps, and a low point as it relaxes. The pressure can be measured using an instrument called a **sphygmomanometer**, and is written as a pair of numbers, such as 120/80. This is the blood pressure of a healthy young adult. Blood pressure increases slowly as we age, and in some people can reach dangerous levels if the proper treatment is not given. When the blood pressure is higher than the normal, the condition is known as **hypertension**.

The body needs to keep the blood under pressure so it can circulate freely all around the body. If blood pressure drops suddenly, as happens when a person suffers "shock" after an accident, the brain and other organs become starved of blood, and the person may lose consciousness.

Blood pressure is measured by a sphygmomanometer. This shows blood pressure by the height of a column of silvery mercury, or by a small dial. The doctor or nurse can tell how tight the sleeve on the arm should be by using the stethoscope to listen to the sound as blood squeezes past the sleeve. Blood pressure can be measured as the heart pumps and between heartbeats.

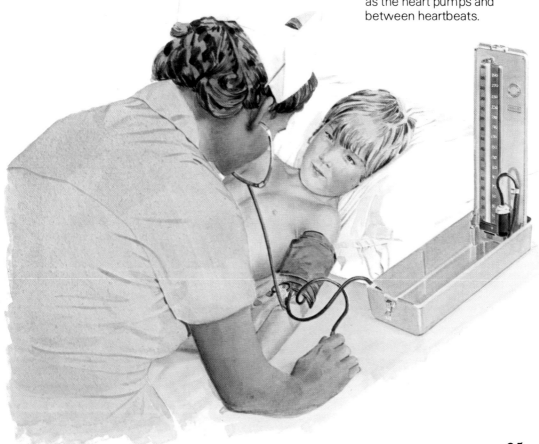

# Red blood cells

Blood is a complicated liquid that contains many special cells as well as important chemicals.

Red cells, or **erythrocytes**, are among the most common. There are 25,000,000,000,000 red cells in the body, each with a life of no more than four months. During this time, they will have traveled around the body in the blood 172,000 times.

In adults, red cells are produced in the spongy marrow inside the largest bones. They are budded off from special cells and carried away in the bloodstream.

Red blood cells are disc-shaped. They have a thin skin or membrane enclosing red jelly-like material which contains hemoglobin. This is the chemical which combines with oxygen so that it can be carried around the body.

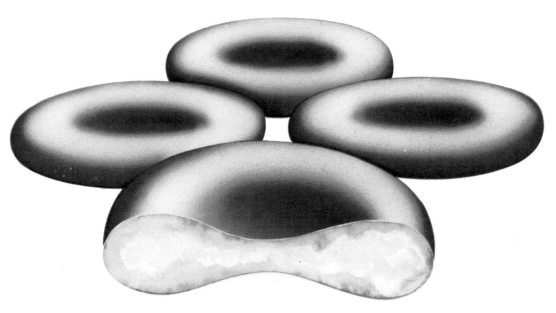

Red cells are shaped like discs, pressed in at the center. They contain large amounts of a chemical called **hemoglobin**, which consists partly of iron. Hemoglobin is a dull purplish-red, giving blood in veins its characteristic dark color.

Hemoglobin is able to combine with oxygen in the lungs to form a new substance, called oxyhemoglobin, which allows the red cells to carry oxygen around the body. When needed by the tissues, the bright red oxyhemoglobin gives up its oxygen and becomes the darker hemoglobin. This is why blood from a cut artery, carrying oxygenated blood, is a much brighter red than that from a vein.

At the end of their short life, red cells are destroyed in the liver, **spleen** and bone marrow, and are replaced by new cells. Each minute 100 million new red cells are made as replacements. Chemicals in the old cells are recycled by the body, some of them being used to make **bile**, which helps in digestion.

# White cells

The other common type of cell in the blood is the white cell, or **leukocyte**.

There are many different types of white cells, each with a special function. There may be 50,000 million in the blood at any one time, and many more during illness.

Their main job is to protect the body by attacking and destroying bacteria and other microbes, and removing or making harmless any foreign substances in the blood, such as those produced by bacteria. They also clear up dead and dying body cells and other waste materials.

As their name suggests, white cells are colorless, and, unlike red cells, they have no special shape. They move about actively, "crawling" along the walls of blood vessels, attacking and eating bacteria by flowing over them.

White cells can squeeze between the cells that make up the thin capillary walls and can roam about in the tissues. Certain types of white cells produce antibodies, chemicals which recognize and link up with foreign material and make it harmless.

The life span of a white cell is only about thirteen to twenty days, and new cells are constantly being formed in the bone marrow, spleen and lymph system.

● white cells made in lymph nodes

❊ red and white cells made in bone marrow

white cells made in liver

Red and white blood cells and platelets are produced in spongy bone marrow, and are carried in the blood around the body. Some types of white blood cell are also produced in the spleen.

Red and white blood cells are made in the bone marrow. White cells are also produced in other parts of the body. The spleen produces red cells for a short while in young babies.

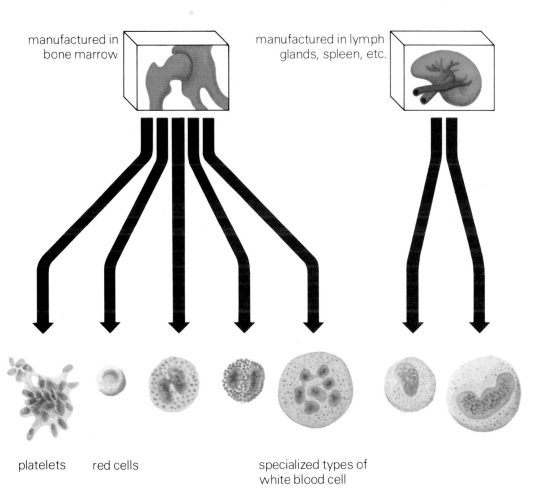

manufactured in bone marrow

manufactured in lymph glands, spleen, etc.

platelets     red cells          specialized types of white blood cell

# Blood plasma

Just over half the blood volume is **plasma**, a straw-colored liquid. Plasma contains other cells, called **platelets**, or **thrombocytes**. These are actually only small parts of cells, nipped off from the tissues that produce them in the bone marrow. Platelets are only a quarter of the size of red cells, and there are many more than the number of red and white cells combined.

The function of platelets is to help the blood to clot after an injury. When cells are damaged, they release substances which react with other chemicals in the plasma and with the platelets to produce long yellow threads of **fibrin**. These form a tangled network in

1 Blood contains platelets, together with chemicals needed for blood clotting.
2 When blood escapes through a wound, more chemicals are released from damaged cells. Platelets begin to congregate in the wound.

fibrin
red blood cells
· platelets

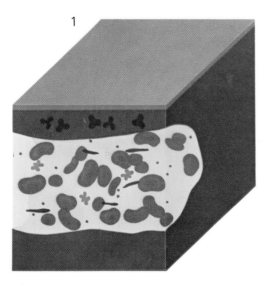
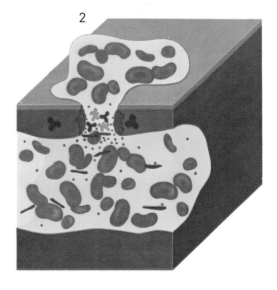

which red and white cells become trapped. After a short while, the fibrin threads shorten, squeezing the whole mass into a hard lump. This is a blood **clot**, or thrombus, which seals the wound while repair is taking place. If the damage is a cut on the skin surface, the clot forms a hard protective scab.

Plasma is mostly water, but it contains an enormous range of dissolved chemicals. **Proteins** in the plasma are used to build and repair cells. Among other substances present are minerals and certain waste materials, such as $CO_2$, on their way to the organs which will eliminate them from the blood.

3 Platelets react with chemicals in the blood and with those released from damaged cells to produce long threads of yellow fibrin, which trap red blood cells.

4 Fibrin threads contract, forming a clot which blocks the wound and prevents further blood loss while healing takes place.

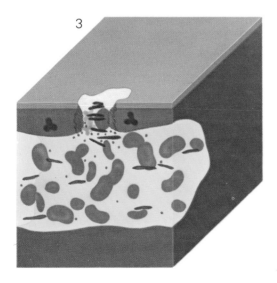

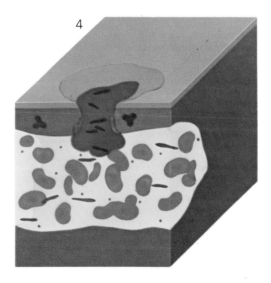

# Fighting disease

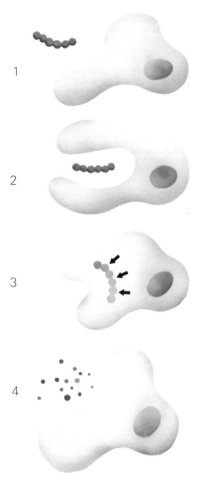

1 A white cell flows toward bacteria like a shapeless blob of jelly.
2 The white cell flows around the string of bacteria.
3 Once inside the white cell, enzymes break down the bacteria.
4 The white cell flows away, leaving behind the undigested remains of the bacteria.

Infections are caused by microscopic organisms which invade the body, usually bacteria or viruses. Some bacteria produce poisons called toxins which damage cells. Viruses are simple organisms which can live inside the body's cells and damage them as they reproduce and emerge.

White blood cells are the main defense against harmful bacteria which enter the body. Bacteria are attacked and consumed by white cells, which travel about in the bloodstream, or are grouped in organs such as the spleen, liver, marrow, or in the lymph system.

The chemicals which make up the protective coat of bacteria are foreign to the body, and are recognized by white cells called **lymphocytes**. When these cells come into contact with this foreign material, they reproduce quickly, and produce a substance called antibody. This enables them to stick to the bacteria and causes the bacteria to group into clumps. They are now immobilized and can be eaten by other white cells.

After the infection has passed, the lymphocytes "remember" how to make the antibody, and can quickly eliminate the same type of bacteria or virus, should they enter the body once more. This is known as a state of **immunity**.

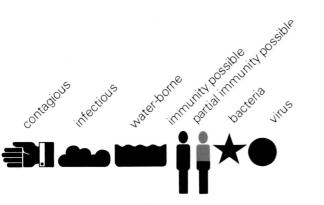

contagious  
infectious  
water-borne  
immunity possible  
partial immunity possible  
bacteria  
virus

The chart below shows some of the most common infectious diseases, how they are spread, and how long it takes for symptoms to appear after having been exposed to the infection.

days

2

4

6

8

10

12

14

16

18

chicken pox  
common cold  
diphtheria  
rubella  
influenza  
measles  
mumps  
polio  
scarlet fever  
whooping cough

33

# Blood groups

Queen Victoria
children
grandchildren
great grandchildren
affected male
female carrier
possible carriers

The body reacts very strongly to most foreign materials which enter the bloodstream. It has little tolerance of some types of blood from other people which might be given as a blood **transfusion** after accident or illness.

If some different types of blood are mixed, chemicals present in the red blood cells and the plasma may react, causing the red cells to stick together, or agglutinate. This can be fatal if a large amount of the wrong type of blood is given in a transfusion.

There are four main types of blood called **blood groups**. These are A, B, AB and O, which is the most common. It is quite safe to receive a transfusion of blood of the same group as your own, and a simple blood test is always given to check on the group whenever a transfusion might be necessary. Group O blood can be given to any of the other groups, except for a few people who have other substances in their blood which could cause problems.

Different races have differing proportions of the four blood groups. South American Indians are entirely Group O, for example, while Asian Indians have a very high proportion of the usually rare Group B.

Blood groups are inherited, like skin, hair and eye color, and are carried in genes

Hemophilia is an inherited disease in which the blood is unable to clot. It affects only males, but women carry the disease and pass it on to their male children. It appeared in Queen Victoria's family and affected many of the crowned families of Europe before dying out.

which control our physical appearance and shape.

In rare cases the blood of the parents of a child contains a combination of **Rhesus (Rh) factors** which cause the mother's blood to damage her unborn baby. A simple blood test now makes this a very uncommon event, and if there is a risk, the baby's blood can be completely changed as soon as it is born.

Hemophilia is a rare inherited disease in which the blood fails to clot. A hemophiliac can bleed badly from a small injury. The disease occurs in certain families, affecting only males, although it is passed on by females who appear healthy.

Blood groups are inherited from genes carried by the parents. In this diagram the first letter shows the person's actual blood group and the second the blood group carried in the genes, which may show up in the offspring. The exception is Group AB, which is a group in its own right.

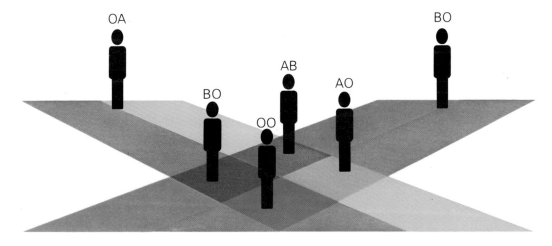

35

# Health problems with the heart and blood

Clotting is a natural function of the blood which reduces blood loss by slowing down bleeding. Clotting can also take place in undamaged blood vessels, probably due to a disturbance in the chemistry of the blood. If the clot breaks away from the wall, it is carried in the bloodstream until it becomes stuck in a narrower blood vessel, which it can block completely.

The blockage cuts off the blood supply to a part of the body, which is then injured and may die. This can happen anywhere in the body, but especially in the brain, where it can cause a **stroke**; in the heart muscle, where it can cause a heart attack; or in the legs.

A more gradual circulatory disease is caused by the gradual blockage of arteries, due to layers of a substance called **cholesterol** being deposited on their walls. The gradual narrowing reduces blood flow to some parts of the body, especially to the heart, where it causes pain called **angina** when the person takes exercise. It can also lead to a heart attack if the arteries narrow sufficiently to cut off the blood flow.

A stroke is damage to the brain, sometimes caused by blockage of a blood vessel with a clot, but more commonly by the bursting of a blood vessel, followed by serious bleeding.

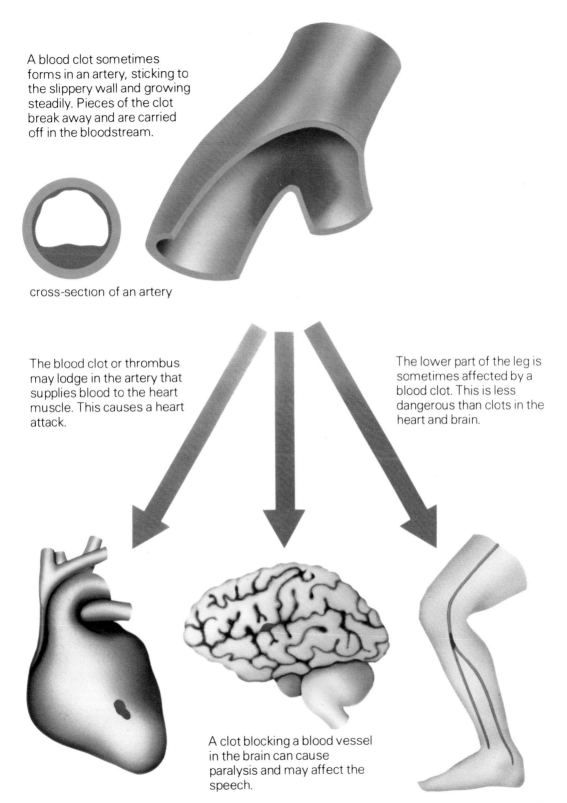

A blood clot sometimes forms in an artery, sticking to the slippery wall and growing steadily. Pieces of the clot break away and are carried off in the bloodstream.

cross-section of an artery

The blood clot or thrombus may lodge in the artery that supplies blood to the heart muscle. This causes a heart attack.

The lower part of the leg is sometimes affected by a blood clot. This is less dangerous than clots in the heart and brain.

A clot blocking a blood vessel in the brain can cause paralysis and may affect the speech.

37

# Heart transplants

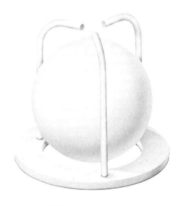

An artificial heart valve is usually a simple "ball in a cage" which moves to allow blood to pass in one direction. It is made of plastic or metal, which will be accepted by the body without causing reactions in the tissue of the heart.

As we age, body organs begin to wear out. Sometimes an organ wears out very rapidly, while the rest of the body is still relatively healthy. When this happens, a replacement, or transplant, operation is sometimes possible. Transplants are never easy, as the body usually tends to attack or reject any strange material put into it.

Heart valves sometimes become damaged by disease, or may even be defective in a newborn baby. This prevents proper blood circulation, and usually can be corrected by replacing the damaged valve with a plastic or metal substitute which the body will accept more readily.

Sometimes the heart muscle is too badly diseased to pump properly, and in rare cases, a heart transplant may be considered. This involves replacing all or part of the heart with one taken from another person, the donor. Donor hearts can only be taken from an accident victim when their brain has permanently stopped working, and they are legally "dead."

The transplant operation itself is not technically difficult, but later there are often complications when the new heart may be rejected. Lifelong drugs are needed to prevent this rejection.

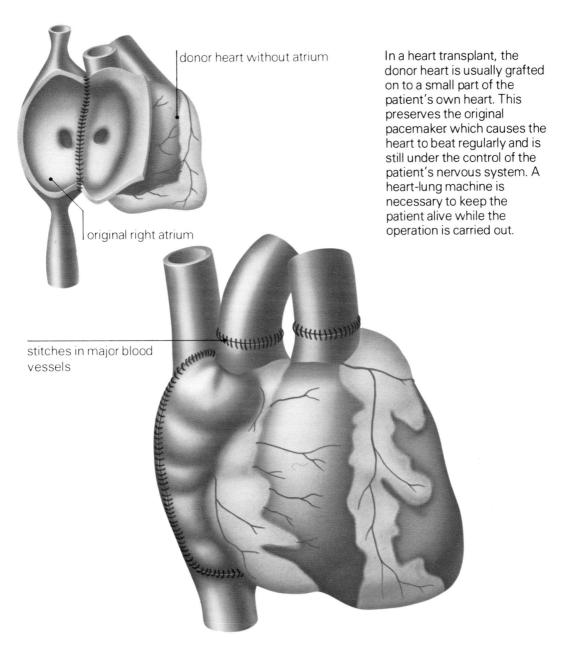

donor heart without atrium

original right atrium

stitches in major blood vessels

In a heart transplant, the donor heart is usually grafted on to a small part of the patient's own heart. This preserves the original pacemaker which causes the heart to beat regularly and is still under the control of the patient's nervous system. A heart-lung machine is necessary to keep the patient alive while the operation is carried out.

Usually the right atrium of the "old" heart is attached to the new heart. This retains the timing mechanism for the heartbeat, and means that the nervous system can still control the new heart, speeding it up during exercise to increase blood flow.

# The lymph system

Blood is under pressure, and plasma can pass freely through the thin walls of the capillaries, passing right through the cells themselves, and also leaking between them. However, the largest molecules cannot pass through, because they are too large for the tiny pores in the cell membranes. Similarly, some protein molecules produced in the tissues outside the capillaries cannot get into the blood, where they are needed.

Plasma leaking into the tissues, together with proteins such as antibodies and enzymes, is collected by a system of ducts called the lymph system. This runs through the body, circulating a clear liquid called **lymph**, which consists of plasma, proteins, and other chemicals. Lymph vessels have a large number of one-way valves, like those in large veins.

Lymph is carried from almost all parts of the body, passing through tiny filters called **lymph nodes**. It eventually flows back into the bloodstream through ducts in the base of the neck.

This recycling of body fluids conserves water and helps to distribute food materials and other essential chemicals to all parts of the body by putting them into the bloodstream.

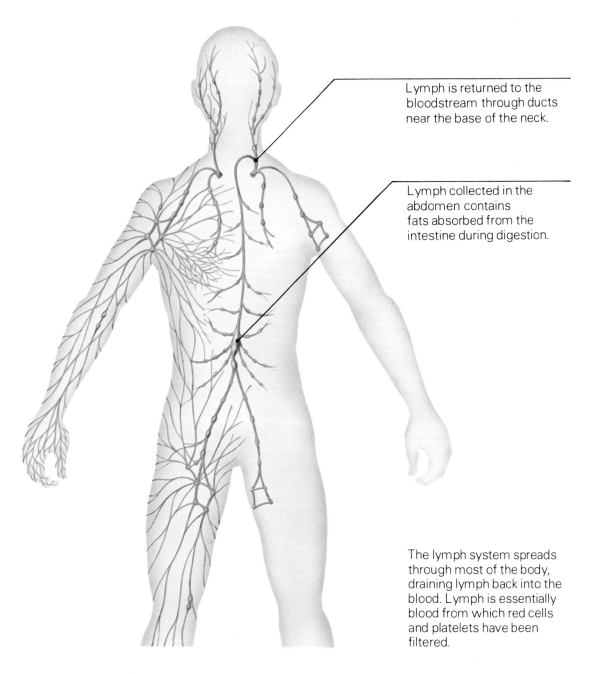

Lymph is returned to the bloodstream through ducts near the base of the neck.

Lymph collected in the abdomen contains fats absorbed from the intestine during digestion.

The lymph system spreads through most of the body, draining lymph back into the blood. Lymph is essentially blood from which red cells and platelets have been filtered.

Lymph also carries large numbers of white cells, or leukocytes. These often pass through capillary walls to the site of an infection, and are later carried away in the lymph to be stored for future use. The lymph system is a major part of the body's defenses against infection.

# The lymph nodes

Lymph nodes (or lymph "glands") are small swellings dotted along the larger lymph vessels. They measure about $\frac{1}{4}$ inch (from 1–10 mm) across and serve to filter the lymph. Most lymph nodes are grouped in the neck, groin, armpits and the lower part of the abdomen.

Inside each node is a spongy mass of tissue through which the lymph flows. Huge numbers of white blood cells, each with a special function, are grouped here.

Loose material floating in the lymph, such as dead cells or bacteria, is consumed by **macrophages**. These are large white cells whose function is to clean up the lymph. Also in the lymph nodes are large numbers of lymphocytes and plasma cells, which produce antibodies against infection and play an important part in developing immunity against infections.

When there is an infection present, the numbers of white cells in the lymph nodes increase enormously, and the nodes may become swollen and tender due to all the activity taking place within them. This is often obvious during an illness, when the "glands" in the side of the neck can be felt with the fingertips.

Other **lymphoid tissue** has a similar

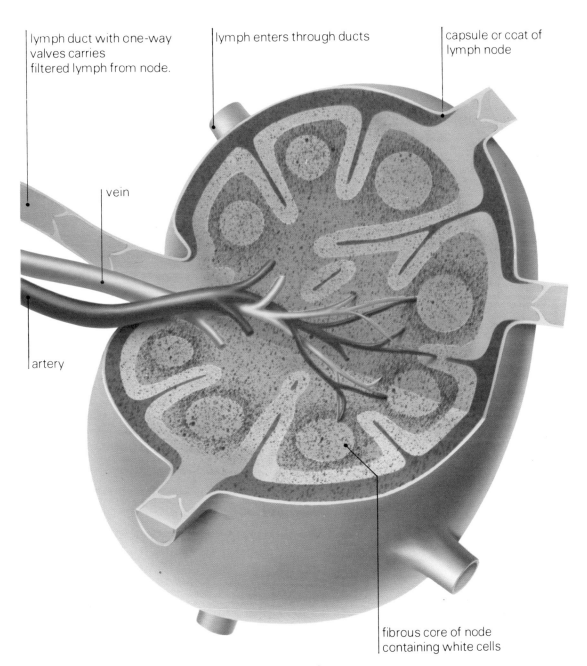

lymph duct with one-way valves carries filtered lymph from node.

lymph enters through ducts

capsule or coat of lymph node

vein

artery

fibrous core of node containing white cells

function to the lymph nodes. Patches of lymphoid tissue are found on the tonsils, adenoids, appendix and throughout the bowel. They function, like the lymph nodes, to filter and destroy bacteria.

The lymph node is an organ for filtering the lymph, removing bacteria, and pouring out antibodies produced by the white cells it contains.

# The spleen

The spleen is a part of the lymph system. It is about 5 inches (125 mm) long, and is positioned on the left side of the lower chest, behind the stomach and above the left kidney.

The spleen contains a mass of red pulp, dotted with small patches of white pulp which make its contents appear grainy. A large amount of blood travels into the spleen, where it first passes through the tiny islands of white pulp. Here there are vast numbers of lymphocytes, which release their antibodies into the blood.

Next the blood passes through an area of special white cells which destroy worn-out red cells and platelets, as well as removing any other solid debris from the blood.

The blood now passes into the red pulp, and back into the circulation. The red pulp may act as a further filter for removing damaged blood cells, but its function is not entirely clear.

In very young babies, the spleen produces red and white blood cells, but it is not essential to life in an adult and can be removed if it becomes diseased.

Like lymph nodes, the spleen becomes swollen and tender during some infections, and its shape can then be felt in the left side just below the ribs.

The spleen is a spongy red organ with a good blood supply. It has important functions in fighting infection, and contains huge numbers of specialized white cells which produce antibodies and consume bacteria and debris in the blood.

The spleen is positioned just below the ribs on the left side of the body toward the back.

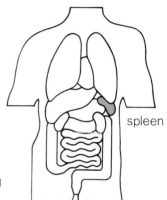

spleen

splenic vein

capsule covering and protecting the spleen

red and white pulp, containing white cells

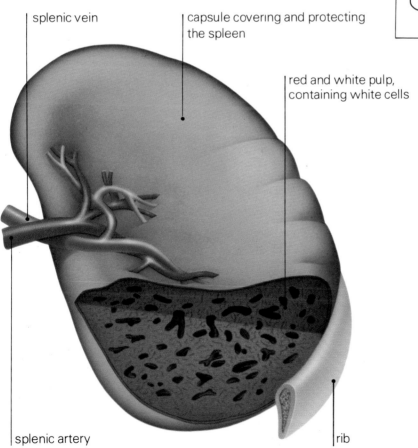

splenic artery

rib

45

# Glossary

**Angina:** severe pain in the chest, caused when arteries supplying blood to the heart muscle become narrowed and the heart is starved of oxygen. It occurs especially during exercise.

**Antibody:** chemical substance produced by white blood cells, which immobilizes disease-producing organisms so they can be destroyed.

**Aorta:** largest artery in the body, receiving blood pumped from the left ventricle.

**Arteriole:** narrow artery, which can become wider or narrower as required, to regulate the blood flow.

**Artery:** vessel carrying blood *away* from the heart. Has a thick, muscular wall to withstand the pressure.

**Atrium:** chamber in the upper part of the heart which receives blood from the body or lungs. There are two atria in the heart. Also sometimes known as the auricle.

**Bile:** greenish substance which helps the body to digest fat. Partly produced by the breakdown of old red blood cells.

**Blood:** liquid containing a wide range of chemicals and special cells, pumped around the body by the heart.

**Blood group:** type of blood which could be safely given as a transfusion to another person within the group. Consists of groups A, B, AB and O.

**Capillaries:** the smallest blood vessels, carrying blood between arteries and veins. Capillary walls are very thin, to allow dissolved materials to pass through.

**Carbon dioxide:** ($CO_2$) colorless gas produced as a waste product by the body. Carried dissolved in the blood, to be removed by the lungs.

**Cardiac muscle:** special types of muscle in the walls of the heart. Its contractions cause the heart to pump.

**Cholesterol:** yellowish fatty substance present in the blood. It may be deposited on the walls of arteries, where it restricts blood flow.

**Circulation:** passage of blood round and round the body.

**Clot:** (or thrombus) forms to prevent blood leaking from a damaged vessel. Clots are produced by chemical reaction between blood factors and platelets. They may sometimes form within an undamaged vessel, and if they break free in the bloodstream, cause blockages elsewhere in the circulation.

**Electrocardiogram:** (ECG) tracing of electrical impulses produced by the heart as it beats. An ECG can show up certain types of heart disease.

**Erythrocyte:** red blood cell.

**Fibrin:** yellow fibers produced by platelets from substances dissolved in the blood. Produces a clot to block a wound.

**Heart:** muscular pump which propels blood around the body, through the system of arteries, capillaries and veins.

**Hemoglobin:** red substance containing iron, found in red blood cells. It combines easily with oxygen, which it carries around the body in the blood.

**Hormones:** chemical messengers, carried in the blood.

**Hypertension:** high blood pressure, which can damage the heart, brain and kidneys if not treated.

**Immunity:** state in which the body resists diseases with which it has previously been infected.

**Leukocyte:** white blood cell.

**Lymph:** liquid from which red blood cells have been filtered, which collects in a special system before passing back into the blood. Important in fighting infection.

**Lymph node:** swelling in the lymph system, where bacteria and other debris are filtered from the lymph.

**Lymphocytes:** white blood cells which produce antibodies in response to an infection.

**Lymphoid tissue:** patches of tissue in the tonsils, adenoids, appendix and parts of the bowel, which filter bacteria from the lymph.

**Macrophage:** white blood cell which consumes bacteria and other debris.

**Oxygen:** colorless gas which is needed by all living cells in the body. It is extracted from the air in the lungs, and carried about the body by hemoglobin in red blood cells.

**Pacemaker:** area in the right atrium which produces electrical impulses that cause the heart to beat regularly. If the natural pacemaker fails, an electronic pacemaker can be fitted surgically.

**Pericardium:** thin bag surrounding the heart. It contains liquid which lubricates the outside of the heart muscle as it pumps.

**Plasma:** clear liquid in which red and white blood cells are suspended. Plasma contains many food materials needed by the body, as well as dissolved wastes.

**Platelets:** (or thrombocytes) small pieces of cell, floating in the blood, which take part in the production of a blood clot to help close a wound.

**Protein:** chemical used to build and repair cells in the body.

**Rhesus factor:** (Rh factor) antigen present on the red blood cells. Certain combinations of Rhesus factor in parents can damage an unborn or newborn baby. Blood transfusions can save an affected baby's life.

**Septum:** strong wall dividing the left and right sides of the heart. A "hole in the heart" is a gap in the septum, allowing oxygenated blood to mix with deoxygenated blood. It can be corrected with surgery.

**Sphygmomanometer:** instrument used to measure blood pressure. An inflatable sleeve is fixed tightly around the upper arm, and pressure is measured on an instrument connected to the sleeve by a tube.

**Spleen:** spongy organ which forms part of the lymph system. It helps the body to fight infection. In babies, the spleen also produces red and white blood cells.

**Stethoscope:** instrument with which a doctor can hear sounds inside the body such as the heartbeat.

**Stroke:** results from the blockage or bursting of a blood vessel in the brain. Damage may be slight or very serious, depending on the part of the brain it affects.

**Thrombocyte:** see Platelets.

**Thrombosis:** blockage of a blood vessel by part of a blood clot or thrombus, causing an area of tissue to be starved of oxygen and die. May cause a stroke or heart attack, and can also cause leg pains.

**Transfusion:** the giving of blood from one person to another. It is necessary to establish the blood group of each person before this can be done safely.

**Varicose veins:** swollen, painful veins, caused by failure of the one-way valves which should prevent blood in the veins from flowing backward down the legs.

**Veins:** thin-walled blood vessels which return blood to the heart.

**Venae cavae:** superior and inferior venae cavae are the largest veins in the body, draining blood directly into the heart.

**Ventricle:** muscular chamber in the heart which pumps blood either to the lungs (right ventricle) or around the body (left ventricle).

# Index

48

-J-
616.

14618
$7.90

The Heart & Blood

## DATE DUE

| | | | |
|---|---|---|---|
| JAN 20 '92 | | | |
| | | | |
| | | | |
| | | | |
| | | | |
| | | | |
| | | | |
| | | | |
| | | | |
| | | | |
| | | | |

DEMCO